Naturally Sweet Delicious

Treats

Trish Blascak

Copyright © 2011 Trish Blascak

All rights reserved.

ISBN: 1466407379
ISBN-13: 978-1466407374

This Book is dedicated to my family and friends, and to those who

want to make a sweet change.

Also to those who want to make a difference regarding the health of

this world.

"Health is the greatest gift, contentment the greatest wealth,
faithfulness the best relationship."
Buddha

CONTENTS

ACKNOWLEDGMENTS

I want to thank everyone who has graced my kitchen during the creation process of these yummy treats. Your taste buds have been invaluable to me!

Thank you also to those who have requested the information that has inspired this book. Such needs cultivated this gift to you.

Thank you to Terry Peyton for taking the time to review this book for publication.

Thank you to everyone who has purchased this book.

Thank you to everyone who will read and use this book.

ABOUT THE AUTHOR

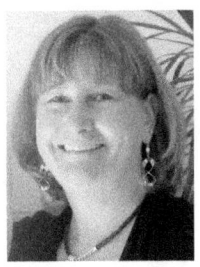

Trish is a holistic health and nutrition educator. She specializes in identifying and treating food sensitivities and provides food sensitivity testing with customized nutritional coaching. Trish is a certified Fitness Nutrition Coach and certified in Reike. She is drawn to homeopathic and holistic means and is versed in EFT, muscle testing, reflexology, Feng Shui, aroma therapy, numerology, herbology, iridology, meditation and yoga. Trish is completing her Master's Degree in Holistic Health and Nutrition Education.

Trish has always loved food and its many aspects from nutrition to shopping to cooking to eating. She is also the author of The Rotation Diet: A New Way of Eating To Promote and Sustain Good Health And Proper Weight. Trish's talents and hobbies of cooking and writing have come together nicely as she currently conducts individual counseling, teaches workshops, performs cooking demonstrations plus continues to write books and articles to promote health and well being.

Trish grew up in Michigan in a busy household with a large family. She is married and has four children and two dogs. Even though her children travel the world, Trish continues to enjoy living in the Great Lakes State of Michigan. Trish enjoys her active family while she continues with her creative, healthy cooking, teaching and writing.

Trish can be contacted through www.myfoodeducation.com.

www.ingramcontent.com/pod-product-compliance
Lightning Source LLC
Chambersburg PA
CBHW060223290526
45789CB00003B/1391

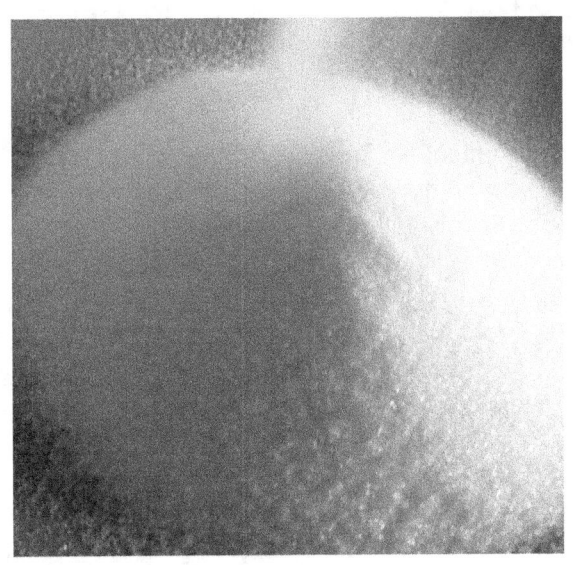

1. SWEET, SWEET SUGAR

Ahh, sugar...sweet, sweet sugar. What a delightful taste on the tongue. What a dreadful effect on the body! How can something that tastes so good, end up being so bad?

The reason is because our bodies were not meant to process large amounts of sugar. It's that Simple! Sugar is a highly processed, non-nutritious, high calorie food that can become addictive. Sugar is a simple carbohydrate and is used by the body for quick energy. If all of the quick energy is not used right away, the body will store the excess energy as fat, for future use. The hormone *insulin* is produced by the body as a part of the sugar metabolism process. If sugar is consumed often, blood insulin levels can fluctuate and be difficult to control. Too much sugar, too often can produce a sustained high insulin level. This in turn can lead to obesity, insulin resistance, hypoglycemia and diabetes. Large amounts of sugar can also lead to food allergies, disturbed hormones, an impaired immune system, dental caries, chronic diseases, heart disease, kidney disease, liver disease, hyperactivity, behavioral problems, inflammatory diseases and an increased risk of cancer, according to Dr. Mercola.

Today the Standard American Diet, otherwise known as SAD, consists of a high amount of animal products, sugar and processed foods and a low amount of fiber, complex carbohydrates and fresh plant-based foods. In contrast, just a few hundred years ago "people mostly consumed fruits, vegetables, wild grains and seeds, fish and occasionally some meat" (Bittman, Mark, 2011). According to Sally Fallon in her book Nourishing Traditions "In 1821, the average sugar intake in America was 10 pounds per person per year, today it is 170 pounds per person per year..." So do we consume too much sugar???

Even though a person may say that they don't eat much sugar, he/she may be getting much more sugar than realized. People may not necessarily indulge in cookies, cakes and ice cream, but sugar has managed to make its way into foods never suspected, that are eaten every day. Foods such as breads, bagels, pizza, French fries, prepared vegetables, canned foods, frozen foods, peanut butter, beverages, dairy products, cereals, chips and snack foods, crackers, processed meats, lunch meats, most sauces such as ketchup, mustard, pizza sauce, mayonnaise, cocktail sauce, salad dressings and spice mixes just to name a few. The sugar in these foods is usually labeled as high fructose corn syrup, corn syrup, fructose, dextrose or sucrose or sometimes...sugar.

Although sugar has been around for at least 2000 years, it was not until the last few hundred years that sugar appeared in the United States. Even at that, it wasn't really until the last 100 years that sugar factories have been a successful commodity. Sugar beet and sugar cane have been the major source of sugar until the 1970's when High Fructose Corn Syrup became popular for its low cost and ease of use. Today, about 750,000,000 bushels of corn per year are used for sweeteners alone. That is equivalent to a cornfield stretching from coast to coast in the United States that is 4 miles wide!!! (www.essortment.com/history-sugar-417)

Sugar is a major business for the US; however, it has some major effects on health. Is it worth it to change the Standard American Diet that so many of us have become accustomed to, towards a healthier diet consisting of less sugar? Try looking at it this way: the definition of a poison is "a substance that through its chemical action kills, injures or impairs an organism" according to Merriam-Webster, http://dictionary.reference.com/browse/poison (n.d.). Wow! Sugar is a substance that through its chemical actions can cause death, injure or impair a person – so is sugar a poison?!!

Knowing all of this, why would anyone ever want to eat sugar? The answer is simple...*knowing* all of this, people probably **wouldn't** want to eat sugar. However, many people don't know the sources of sugary foods or what sugar does to the body. Information is knowledge and knowledge is power. An informed person has the power to decide what is best, and then choose accordingly.

The good news is that there are many natural alternatives to sugar. These alternative still provide the satisfaction of sweetness, however, they offer various other benefits as well. Some natural alternative sweeteners provide vitamins and minerals while others may have a sweet taste but don't elevate the insulin level (considered a low glycemic food). Yet others have additional health benefits such as reducing tooth decay or enhancing the immune system. And still others can provide the sweetness we sometimes desire, but offer zero calories.

As your palate becomes more familiar with these natural alternative sweeteners, you may develop a favorite or two. Just remember that regardless of where it comes from...*sweets are treats* and are **not** meant to be eaten all day long, every day. However, it is nice to know that when you do want to indulge in a special treat – you can do so without feeling guilty!

A word about artificial sweeteners

There has been much controversy as to whether artificial sweeteners are acceptable for human consumption or not. Artificial sweeteners are chemical compounds that have a sweet taste. They are not found in nature and are not natural to our bodies. Our bodies view these chemicals as invaders and try to eliminate them, sometimes causing serious damage to the body. Many books and articles have been written based on human and animal studies conducted on artificial sweeteners. Research shows that artificial sweeteners can cause some serious side effects such as headaches, dizziness, nausea, vision changes, fatigue, weakness, convulsions, hives, rashes, diarrhea, sleep problems, stuffy nose, runny nose, red and itchy eyes, bloating, gas, vomiting, heart palpitations, joint pains and aches, anxiety, panic, anger and depression to name a few (Mercola, 2006).

I urge you to stay away from all artificial sweeteners.

Please note: I have found one good use for artificial sweeteners. Because these chemicals have damaging effects on the nervous system, I sprinkle a few packets of artificial sweetener (aspartame works the best) by my back door to eliminate my spring ant problem!

Naturally Sweet Delicious Treats

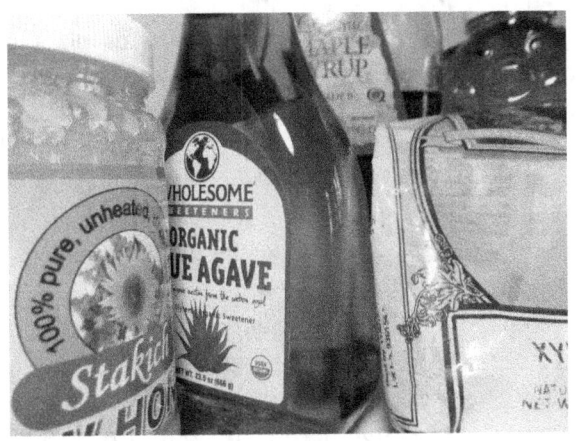

2. SUGAR ALTERNATIVES

When cane sugar or beet sugar is not an option, there are other natural sweeteners to consider. The key here is 'natural' sweeteners, not 'artificial' sweeteners. Artificial sweeteners are chemicals that the body is not built for, therefore posing possible issues for future health (even though many artificial sweeteners have been approved by the FDA, several health issues have surfaced from continued use of these chemicals).

Sugar alternatives:

*Agave – such as organic blue agave or organic raw agave. This can be found in most grocery stores and health food stores. Agave syrup or nectar is made from a cactus plant native to Mexico called the Agave plant. This is a *low glycemic* sweetener that is sweeter than table sugar, so a lesser amount is needed compared to that of table sugar. Agave is a syrup that does not crystallize in the bottle over time, yet dissolves easily in hot or cold liquids. Agave helps retain moisture in foods so it is great for baking because it increases the shelf life of a product.

*Stevia – comes in a liquid or powder form and is about 150 to 400 times sweeter than sugar (depending on the brand – look for pure Stevia). Stevia can be found in health food stores and most grocery stores. Stevia is an herb from South America where the leaves have been used as a sweetener for hundreds of years. Some of the powder forms of Stevia seem to have a slight bitter aftertaste, but most liquids do not. Liquid Stevia is good for beverages and the powder is better for baking. However, Stevia does not substitute well for sugar in all recipes because so little is needed which changes the consistency of the finished baked good. Keep in mind that when using Stevia it *can actually lower blood sugar levels*, so don't use it when/if you are hypoglycemic.

*Xylitol – is a granulated powder that can be found in most health food stores. Xylitol is made from the bark of birch trees and has 40% less calories than table sugar. It is metabolized in the body without the use of insulin, so it is a *low glycemic* food. Xylitol has many health benefits but is mostly known for the prevention of tooth decay and gum disease. Xylitol has been used in the United States as a food ingredient (especially chewing gums) since the 1960's. It can be substituted equally for sugar.

Barley Malt Syrup – is a liquid sweetener, much like molasses. This can be found at health food stores and some local grocery stores. This sweetener is made from sprouted barley which is cooked down to a syrup. Even though this syrup is about half as sweet as table sugar and the body metabolizes it more slowly than table sugar, *it can still raise glycemic levels* due to the carbohydrate content. Otherwise barley malt syrup is a great sweetener for baking and sauces because of its wholesome or 'nutty' flavor.**

Brown Rice Syrup – is a liquid sweetener, much like honey. This can be found at health food stores and some local grocery stores. This sweetener is made from fermented brown rice which is then boiled down to a syrup. It metabolizes more slowly than table sugar however *it can still raise glycemic levels* due to the carbohydrate content. Otherwise, brown rice syrup is a great whole food sweetener to use for baking and in hot drinks.**

Date Sugar – is a very sweet natural sugar that can be found in health food stores and some local grocery stores. Date sugar is made from dehydrated dates that are ground into a powder. Fresh, whole dates are considered a low glycemic food however; when dates are dehydrated they become very concentrated and very sweet, thus being considered *a high glycemic food*. Date sugar is high in fiber as well as vitamins and minerals since it is a whole food. It does not dissolve well in liquids but is great for baking.

Honey – is a very sweet liquid – twice as sweet as sugar so use it sparingly. Honey can be found in most stores and raw honey can be found in most health food stores and some grocery stores. Honey is very sweet so it is considered a *high glycemic* food. Bees make honey from flower nectar. It takes one bee an entire lifetime to make one tablespoon of honey. Most of us are accustomed to processed honey, which has been heated and filtered to remove bee pollen, however when honey is processed it loses enzymes, vitamins and minerals. On the other hand *raw* honey is loaded with enzymes and some vitamins and minerals. Honey will crystallize over time, but can be liquefied by placing the jar in warm water for 10-15 minutes. Honey has many health benefits if used in its raw state (see important note below regarding raw honey and infants). I use honey for much of my baking, to sweeten drinks and to top toast for a sweeter taste.

Maple Syrup or Maple sugar – is a very sweet liquid or crystal so use it sparingly. This can be found in health food stores and local grocery stores. Real maple syrup is made from collecting the sap of maple trees and boiling it down to a syrup. Maple sugar is crystallized maple syrup. Maple syrup or maple sugar is considered a **high glycemic** food and is metabolized much like table sugar. This is a great unprocessed, natural sweetener to use for baking or in hot or cold liquids.

Fruit Spreads – natural fruit spreads are a good alternative for jellies and jams. Make sure the label does not list any added sugar – it should be fruit sweetened only. Fruit spreads can be found in health food stores and some local grocery stores. I use fruit spreads to top my toast, for peanut butter and "jelly" sandwiches and to sweeten pancakes or smoothies.

Rapadura – is dehydrated cane sugar juice. Rapadura contains the molasses as well as the full spectrum of nutrients of the whole sugar cane, because it is not a refined product. Therefore this is considered a healthier choice than refined white sugar, but again, too much Rapadura can have some of the same negative effects on the body as refined sugar.

New sweeteners are being introduced in the market place at a rapid rate. It can be difficult and confusing to choose one that is right for you. Choose sweeteners that are natural and not chemically altered. Make sure that nothing has been 'added' to the natural sweetener (which could change its effect on the body). Marketing experts can make a poison sound like a tempting, luxurious treat - so be a wise consumer!

"What is food to one man may be fierce poison to others."
Lucretius

*indicates low glycemic

** If you are sensitive to monosodium glutamate (MSG), this sweetener *should not* be used because it is made from a fermented product.

Important Note regarding raw honey and infants:

The American Academy of Pediatrics advises that raw or unpasteurized honey should be avoided by infants and children under 12 months of age.

Trish Blascak

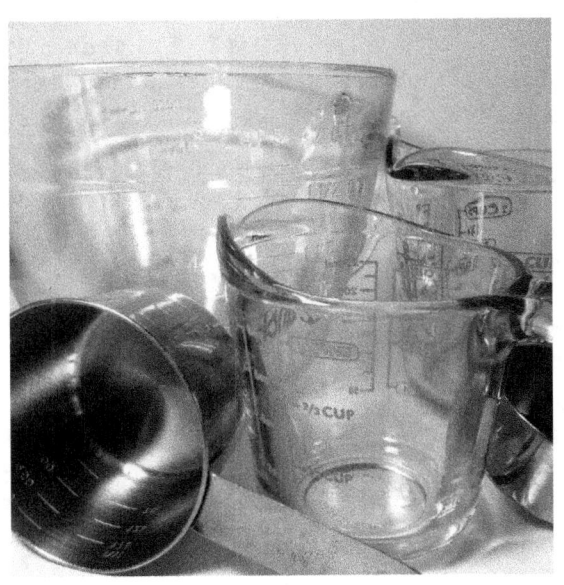

3. SUGAR SUBSTITUTIONS

The following sugar substitutions are equivalent replacements for 1 cup of white granulated sugar. Keep in mind that all sweeteners do not substitute equally, so other actions may be needed to equalize sugar.

If you do not find a suitable substitution, it is possible to limit your sugar intake in baked goods by reducing the total amount of sugar called for in a recipe by half. In addition to this reduction you might want to enhance the overall flavor of the baked good by doubling the amount of vanilla or other extract flavorings in the recipe. If no extract is called for - add 1 tsp vanilla extract or 1/2 tsp cinnamon to enhance the 'sweetness' of the baked good using the appropriate flavors accordingly.

Agave   ¾ cup agave = 1 cup sugar. Also slightly reduce the amount of other liquid in the recipe and reduce the oven temperature by 25 degrees.

Stevia   ½ teaspoon powder Stevia = 1 cup sugar
           1 teaspoon liquid Stevia = 1 cup sugar

Because Stevia has no bulk, add a ⅓ cup of liquid bulk such as: yogurt, applesauce, fruit juice, egg whites or water.

Xylitol   1 cup Xylitol = 1 cup sugar. Even though this substitution is 1 to 1, Xylitol has 40% less calories than sugar.

Barley Malt Syrup   1⅓ cups barley malt syrup = 1 cup sugar. Also reduce the amount of other liquid by ¼ cup.

Brown Rice Syrup   1¼ cup brown rice syrup = 1 cup sugar. Also reduce the amount of other liquid by ¼ cup.

Date Sugar   1 cup date sugar = 1 cup sugar (brown or white).

Honey   ¾ cup honey = 1 cup sugar. Reduce the amount of other liquid by ¼ cup and reduce the oven temperature by 25 degrees.

Maple Syrup   ¼ cup maple syrup = 1 cup sugar. Also reduce the amount of other liquid by 3 tablespoons.

Fruit Spreads   no exact substitution. I use a 1 to 1 substitution but only in small amounts.

Rapadura   1 cup of Rapadura = 1 cup refined white sugar.

Naturally Sweet Delicious Treats

Trish Blascak

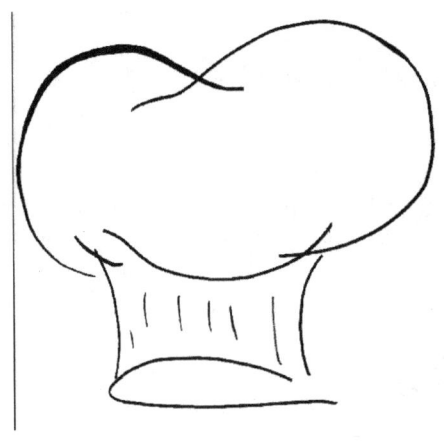

4. RECIPES

The following is a collaboration of recipes that have been created for those "sweet" times. There are some definite favorites that are "must have" treats in my house. Let your inner chef discover some of your own favorites to add to your collection of traditions!

Feel free to play around with each recipe as your creative side desires. Add a little love and it will always turn out magnificent!

"I feel a recipe is only a theme, which an intelligent cook can play each time with a variation."
Madam Benoit

Almond Butter Cookies

Makes 3 dozen cookies
These are completely sugar free and low glycemic. These cookies
taste great with tea, coffee or milk.

1 cup organic butter – softened
½ cup agave syrup
1 tsp vanilla extract
2 tsp almond extract
1 tbsp organic orange juice
2 ½ cups organic whole wheat flour
2 tsp baking powder
½ tsp Stevia powder

Preheat oven to 400°. Spray cookie sheet with cooking spray and set aside.

In a mixing bowl beat butter and agave until fluffy. Add the vanilla, almond and orange juice and mix well. Next add the flour, baking powder and Stevia powder and mix well until dough forms. Make 1" balls and place on cookie sheet. Press each ball with the bottom of a glass cup and flatten to about 1/8 inch thickness. For fancier cookies, press with a cup that has a design on the bottom to imprint the cookie dough, or use a cookie press.

Bake for 6-8 minutes – until slightly brown around the edges. Place on wire rack to cool.

Carrot Cake

Makes one 9x13 cake
This is an eggless, dairy free cake that is actually 'good' for
you...just don't tell the kids - they'll never know how healthy this
treat really is!

1 ¼ cups organic carrots - chopped
1 banana
1 cup organic apple sauce - no sugar added
1 cup vegetable oil
1 tsp apple cider vinegar
2 cups organic whole wheat flour
1 tsp baking soda
2 tsp baking powder
½ tsp salt
2 tsp cinnamon
½ tsp ground cloves
¼ tsp ground nutmeg
⅛ tsp ground ginger

Preheat oven to 325°. Prepare a 9x13 baking pan by spraying
with cooking spray. Set aside until ready to use.

Put the carrots in a sauce pan and cover with water. Bring to a
boil and cook, covered until soft - about 10 minutes. Drain water
and mash carrots by hand, with a fork or in the blender, on
medium, until only slightly chunky. Set aside to cool slightly.
Meanwhile, in a mixing bowl mash the banana with a fork then
add the apple sauce, vegetable oil and apple cider vinegar. Mix in
the mashed carrots and blend well. In a separate bowl add the
flour, baking soda, baking powder, salt, cinnamon, cloves, nutmeg
and ginger and whisk together. Carefully mix the wet ingredients
into the dry ingredients. Pour batter into prepared 9x13 pan.
Bake at 325° for 30-40 minutes. Let cake cool slightly. Serve as is
or with 'No Sugar Frosting' - recipe on page 33.

Cherry Bars

Makes 20 bars
These make a fantastic energy bar as well as being a delicious treat.

1 cup raw almonds
½ cup dried cherries
1 cup pitted dates
1 tsp vanilla extract
½ tsp almond extract
¼ cup water

Preheat oven to 180°. Spray a cookie pan (15' X 10') with cooking spray and set aside.

Place all ingredients in blender or food processor and blend for about 1-2 minutes – until mixture is blended, but still chunky. Carefully press mixture, evenly, into greased cookie pan, beginning in the center and working your way out to the edges. It may be helpful to wet your fingers with water so that the mixture doesn't stick to your hands.

Place cherry bars in the oven for 4-6 hours to dehydrate. When desired hardness is reached, remove from oven and let cool about 15 minutes. Cut into bars and let cool completely. Remove from cookie sheet and serve, or put in airtight container. These bars will keep in the refrigerator for up to two weeks.

Chocolate Cheese Cake

Makes 8-10 servings
This is a quick, easy recipe you can prepare in the microwave.
What a great idea for those leftover brownies!

Crust:
¼ cup organic butter - melted
1 tbsp Agave
1 ½ cup brownie crumbs (brownie recipe on page 26)

Filling:
8 oz organic cream cheese - softened
1 organic egg
2 tbsp raw honey
1 tsp vanilla extract
1 tbsp cocoa

Topping:
1 cup organic sour cream
1 tbsp honey

Mini chocolate chips or cocoa powder for garnish - optional.

To prepare the crust put melted butter, agave and brownie crumbs in a bowl and mix well. Wet fingers and pat mixture into a glass pie pan, working some of the crust slightly up the edges of the pan. Set aside.

For the filling put the cream cheese in a bowl then add the egg, honey vanilla and cocoa and beat until smooth. Pour filling into crust and cook on high in microwave for 2 minutes. Turn pan then cook for another 2 minutes.

To make topping put the sour cream in a glass measuring cup and microwave on high for 25 seconds to soften. Add the honey and mix well. Carefully pour over the partially cooked filling, starting at the outer edges first (center will still be soft). Return to microwave and cook for 1-2 minutes more – until no longer soft in the middle. Let cool slightly then garnish with chocolate chips or cocoa. Refrigerate for at least 2 hours until well set. Serve cold.

Chocolate Fudge

Makes 16 pieces
This fudge is best served nice and cold straight from the refrigerator.

1 cup pitted dates
1 cup raw cashews
2 tbsp cocoa powder or Cacao powder*
1 tbsp coconut oil
2 tbsp Agave
3 tbsp water

Put all ingredients in blender or food processor and process on high until smooth consistency (2-4 minutes). Let mixture rest in blender or food processor for about 20 minutes. Next, scoop mixture into greased 8x8 pan and cover with plastic wrap. Place fudge in refrigerator for several hours or overnight. Cut into squares and serve cold.

*Cacao powder is a Mayan superfood. It is raw chocolate powder that is loaded with healthy antioxidants, iron and magnesium. This can be found in most health food stores.

Cinnamon Rolls

Makes 12 servings
There is nothing like the sweet smell of cinnamon drifting throughout the house as these treats are baking! This is a favorite treat in my house.

Dough:
¾ cup organic milk
3 tbsp organic butter
2 tbsp raw honey
3 ½ - 4 cups whole wheat flour
2 pkg yeast (¼ oz each)
1 tsp sea salt
1 organic egg
½ cup organic sour cream

Filling:
¼ cup organic butter
⅓ cup Agave
2 tbsp cinnamon

Put milk and butter in microwave safe bowl and heat for 2 minutes on high. Add the honey and stir. Set aside.

Mix 1 ½ cups of the flour, yeast, egg and sour cream together. Add the warm milk mixture and whisk until smooth. Add enough remaining flour to make dough. You may need to mix with a spoon at first and then your hands. Turn dough onto a floured surface and gather into a ball. Knead by pressing the heel of your hand firmly into the dough, pushing forward slightly. Fold the edges of the dough into the center and rotate dough slightly. Repeat with this press, fold and turn sequence for 3-5 minutes, adding additional flour as needed to prevent stickiness. The dough should be smooth and elastic at this point. Put 2 tbsp. of vegetable oil into a bowl swirling to coat sides of bowl. Place the dough in the bowl turning to coat all sides with the oil. Cover with plastic wrap and put the bowl in a warm place (about 70° to 85°) and let the dough rise for 15-30 minutes - until doubled in size.

To make filling, place butter in a microwave safe bowl and microwave for 40 seconds to melt. Add the agave and cinnamon and whisk until smooth. Set aside.

Once the dough has doubled in size, remove the plastic cover, punch dough down to release air bubbles and place dough ball on clean counter or table. The oil that is already on the dough should be sufficient for rolling - no need to flour the counter. Roll out dough with a rolling pin into a 12 x 18 rectangle. Using a spatula or the back of a spoon, spread filling evenly over dough, making sure to spread all the way to the edges. Roll dough - long ways in a jelly roll fashion, to form an 18" log shape. Pinch edges and ends tightly to seal, folding in ends. Slice into 12 even pieces and place on greased cookie pan (15" X 10") - cut side up. Cover with a towel and let rise for 15-30 minutes in warm place (70° to 85°). Bake at 350° for 15-20 minutes. Frost with 'no sugar frosting'- recipe on page 33.

*hint – dough will rise quickly if you turn oven on to 180° for 5 minutes **then turn off**. Place covered dough in closed (turned off) oven to rise.

Delightful Brownies

Makes about 20 brownies
The Xylitol in these brownies leaves a clean, fresh taste in your mouth afterwards. What a delightful benefit from a sweet treat!

½ cup organic butter
½ cup cocoa powder
3 tbsp water
1 cup Xylitol
1 organic egg
1 tsp vanilla extract
1 cup organic whole wheat flour

Preheat oven to 350°.

Put butter in microwave safe bowl and melt in microwave – about 45 seconds. Add the cocoa, water and Xylitol and mix well. Next add the egg and vanilla and mix well. Add the flour and mix until batter forms. Pour into a greased 9x9 square pan or a 10" round pan. Bake for 15-20 minutes – until toothpick comes out clean. Be careful not to over bake or the brownie will be dry. Spread with glaze (see recipe below.)

Glaze
2 tbsp organic butter
1 tbsp potato starch
2 tbsp Xylitol
½ tbsp cocoa powder

Put butter in small bowl and melt in microwave. Add the potato starch, Xylitol and cocoa powder. Mix well with whisk. Spread evenly over brownies. Serve.

Eggless, Sugarless Banana Bread

Makes 3 small loaves or 1 large loaf
The smell of fresh banana bread warms a home! This is a truly simple, delicious, healthy way to indulge.

3-4 ripe bananas
½ cup honey
½ cup canola oil
1 ½ cup organic whole wheat flour
1 tsp baking soda
½ tsp salt

Preheat oven to 400°.

Prepare loaf pans by spraying with cooking spray. Set aside.

Peel and mash bananas in a mixing bowl, with a fork or potato masher. Add the honey and oil. Mix until well combined and almost creamy. Add the flour, baking soda and salt and mix until just combined.

Put batter into prepared loaf pans and bake at 400° for 30-45 minutes. Toothpick should come out clean when done. Do not over bake or the bread will be dry.

Cool on a wire rack for at least 10 minutes before serving.

Fruit Dip

Makes about 1 cup
This is a great dip for fresh berries, apples, grapes, sliced bananas,
pineapples or other fresh fruit.

8 oz organic cream cheese – softened
½ cup raw honey
1 tsp vanilla extract

Put all ingredients in blender and whip on high, until smooth and
fluffy, about 1-2 minutes. Put in a serving bowl, cover and chill
until ready to use.

Graham Cookies

Makes about 3 dozen cookies
These eggless cookies have a slightly sweet taste with a nice buttery after-taste. They are wonderful with tea or coffee. Variations of this cookie are sure to entertain the palate.

1 cup organic butter - softened
½ cup black strap molasses
¼ cup raw honey
3 ½ cups whole grain graham flour
½ tsp sea salt
1 tsp baking soda
1 tsp baking powder
1 tsp cinnamon

Preheat oven to 350°.

Cream together the butter, molasses and honey. Then add the flour, salt, baking soda, baking powder and cinnamon. Mix well. Drop by teaspoon onto greased cookie sheet. Bake for 10-12 minutes. Let cool slightly on cookie sheet then transfer to wire rack to continue cooling.

Variations:

Ginger Cookie - use ½ tsp ground ginger instead of cinnamon

Spice Cookie - add ½ tsp ground ginger and ¼ tsp each of ground cloves and ground nutmeg along with the cinnamon.

Trish Blascak

Magnificent Stovetop Granola

Makes 6 servings
This is a soft or chewy granola rather than the more traditional crunchy version.

4 tbsp organic butter
1 cup organic oats
3 tbsp raw honey
¼ tsp cinnamon

Melt butter in large skillet. When butter is melted, add the oats and mix to coat. Add the honey and cinnamon and mix well. Cook on medium-high, stirring often, until toasted - about 3-5 minutes. Turn granola out onto a plate to cool. Break apart into bite size pieces and enjoy!

Feel free to add additions to this granola such as almonds, pecans, raisins or dried cranberries. Add any of these ingredients to the skillet with the other ingredients and cook as directed above.

If you choose to add chocolate chips - do so after the granola cools. Do not add chocolate chips to the skillet - they will melt!

Muffins

Makes 18 regular muffins or 48 mini muffins
These muffins are sweetened naturally with honey, agave and
blueberries. They are great for breakfast or a snack.

½ cup organic butter
⅓ cup raw honey
1 tbsp Agave
⅔ cup organic sour cream
2 tsp vanilla extract
2 cups organic whole wheat flour
2 tsp baking soda
½ tsp sea salt
1 (16 oz) bag of frozen organic blueberries (about 2 ½ cups -
frozen)

Preheat oven to 350° Prepare muffin tins by spraying them with
cooking spray.

Put frozen blueberries in microwave safe bowl and defrost for 2
minutes on high. They will be very juicy at this point, that's ok, it
helps to flavor the muffins. Set aside.

In a separate bowl cream together the butter, honey, agave, sour
cream and vanilla. Then add the flour baking soda and salt. Mix
together. Add the blueberries and stir just to mix. Fill each
muffin tin about ⅔ full.

Bake as follows:
                    Mini muffins - 12-15 minutes
                    Regular muffins - 15-20 minutes

Toothpick should come out clean when inserted. Let muffins cool
for 5 minutes in tins, then transfer to wire rack to continue to
cool. (Variations on next page)

Muffin variations: use different fruits in place of the blueberries:

Cherry: 2 ½ cups frozen cherries - plus add ½ tsp almond extract

Apple: 2 ½ cups diced, fresh apples - plus ½ tsp cinnamon and ¼ cup applesauce

No Sugar Frosting

Makes about 1 cup
This frosting is great for carrot cake, cinnamon rolls or any other reason you may need frosting! This is a fantastic sugar free alternative.

4 oz organic cream cheese - softened
4 tbsp organic butter - softened
3 tbsp Agave syrup
4 tbsp of potato starch
2 tsp vanilla extract
Up to 2 tbsp organic milk - as needed

Cream together the butter and cream cheese with an electric mixer or by hand with a whisk. Beat in the Agave syrup and vanilla. Then beat in the potato starch. Add enough milk for desired consistency and beat well. If frosting gets too runny, add a little bit more potato starch and/or put frosting in refrigerator to thicken. Spread accordingly on baked goods.

Oatmeal Cherry Cookies

Makes 3 ½ dozen cookies
These are good, wholesome cookies made with no sugar. They make a great hearty snack or wholesome breakfast coupled with a glass of milk.

1 cup organic butter - softened
4 tbsp raw honey
¼ cup Agave syrup
2 tsp vanilla extract
2 organic eggs
2 ½ cups organic whole wheat flour
½ tsp baking soda
¼ tsp sea salt
1 cup organic oats
1 ½ cups dried cherries
½ cup chopped pecans (optional)

Preheat oven to 325°.

Cream together the butter, honey, Agave syrup, vanilla and eggs. Add the flour, baking soda, salt and oats and mix until dough forms. Mix in the cherries and pecans. Drop cookies by tablespoon on greased cookie sheet. Bake for 11-14 minutes. Remove from oven and let cool slightly, then transfer to wire rack to cool completely. Store in airtight container.

Peaches and Cream

Makes 4-6 servings
This is a wonderful comfort food with all the fuzzy feelings of
home and completely sugar free and diary free!

5 organic peaches
1 cup raw almonds
1½ cups water
½ tsp almond extract (optional)

Wash peaches and carefully cut into cubes (I leave the skin on but
you may peel it if you prefer). Place peaches in bowl and
refrigerate until ready to serve.

Put almonds and water into blender. Blend on high for about 2-3
minutes, until mixture is very smooth. Add the almond extract, if
you are using it, and blend. Now pour the 'almond cream' into a
small serving pitcher and place in refrigerator until ready to use.

To serve, place some diced peaches in a small bowl and drizzle
almond cream on top. Enjoy!

If the peaches are a little bit tart - you may add 1-2 tbsp of Agave
or raw honey to the almond cream and serve as above.

Peanut Butter Balls

Makes 12 balls
Peanut Butter and chocolate, what a great combination!
Sometimes I serve these with breakfast!

½ cup organic peanut butter
½ cup brown rice syrup
2 tbsp organic butter – softened
1 tbsp potato starch
1- 3.5 oz organic dark chocolate bar *

In a bowl mix together the peanut butter, brown rice syrup and softened butter until smooth and creamy. Add the potato starch and mix well. Put mixture in the refrigerator for about 1 hour, until mixture is firm enough to form into balls.

Remove mixture from refrigerator and form into 12 balls. Place on waxed paper covered cookie sheet, and place in freezer for at least 1 hour.

Meanwhile, break apart organic chocolate bar and place pieces in a small microwave safe bowl. Melt chocolate at 70% power for 1-3 minutes, until chocolate is melted and smooth, mixing half way through. Set aside.

Remove peanut butter balls from the freezer. Dip each ball into the melted chocolate, swirling around to cover entire ball. Place back on waxed paper. Chocolate should harden quickly on the cold peanut butter. Serve when chocolate has set.

* The darker the chocolate the less sugar it contains. I prefer 75% to 85% cacao. Choose an organic bar that uses Rapadura or unrefined organic sugar such as *Rapunzel* organic dark chocolate bar, or *Green and Black's* Organic dark chocolate bar.

Peanut Butter Torte

Makes 1 torte – about 12 servings
This delicious torte finishes a meal charmingly and is gluten free
and egg free.

Prepare a springform pan by spraying with cooking spray. Set aside.

For crust:
½ cup raw almonds
¾ cup raisins
3 tbsp organic butter
1 tsp vanilla extract
A pinch of coriander
1 cup raw sesame seeds
1 tbsp Agave
2-3 tbsp raw honey

Put almonds, raisins, butter, vanilla, coriander, sesame seeds, agave and raw honey in blender. Blend until mixture becomes pasty. You may need to add 1-2 tbsp of water if necessary for blending. Using a spatula or back of a spoon, spread the paste in the bottom of the prepared springform pan, working up the edge a bit to form a small crust.

Place pan in the refrigerator to set, while preparing the filling.

For Filling:
2 cups raw cashews
1 cup water
1 cup organic peanut butter (or natural with no added sugars)
¼ cup organic butter – melted and cooled
2 tbsp vanilla extract
2 tbsp agave
½ tbsp fresh lemon juice

⅓ cup raw honey
¼ cup of brown rice flour

Place the cashews, water, peanut butter, melted butter, vanilla, agave, lemon juice and honey in the blender. Mix until nuts are smooth and creamy. Pour the mixture into a bowl and stir in rice flour.

Remove the pan with the crust from the refrigerator. Carefully pour the filling over the crust and smooth out with a spatula. You may sprinkle the top with dark chocolate chips, chocolate shavings, chopped peanuts or drizzle with organic, dark chocolate syrup.

Return torte to the refrigerator for at least 4-6 hours before serving.

Enjoy!

Pumpkin Muffins

Makes 12 muffins
You can infuse the mood of "Autumn" any time of the year with
these delicious, aromatic muffins!

1 16 oz can of organic pumpkin
⅓ cup organic, natural applesauce
½ cup Rapadura
2 tbsp raw honey
½ cup canola oil
1 ½ cups organic whole wheat flour
1 tsp baking soda
½ tsp salt
½ tsp baking powder
2 tsp cinnamon
¼ tsp ground ginger
¼ tsp nutmeg
¼ tsp cloves
2 tbsp Rapadura for topping

Preheat oven to 350°. Prepare muffin tins by spraying with
cooking spray. Set aside.

In a bowl, add pumpkin, applesauce, Rapadura, honey and oil.
Mix until well blended and creamy. Add the flour, baking soda,
salt, baking powder, cinnamon, ground ginger, nutmeg and
cloves. Stir until just mixed. Fill each muffin tin about ¾ full.
Sprinkle the tops of each muffin with the remaining 2 tbsp of
sugar – topping all 12 muffins.

Bake at 350° for 20-25 minutes or until toothpick comes out
clean. Do not over bake.

Serve warm or cool completely and store in airtight container.

Stovetop Granola

Makes 6 servings
This makes a great 'munchy' to put out for a special occasion or to top off yogurt for a special treat.

4 tbsp organic butter
1 cup organic oats
3 tbsp maple syrup
½ cup slivered almonds

Melt butter in large skillet. When butter is melted, add the oats and mix to coat. Add the maple syrup and mix well. Cook for about 1 minute then add the almonds. Cook on medium-high, stirring often, until oats and almonds are toasted - about 3-5 minutes. Turn granola out onto a plate to cool. Break apart into bite size pieces and enjoy!

Strawberry Chocolate Mousse

Makes 4 servings
You can fool all your friends with this delicious, fluffy mousse.
They'll never guess it's made from avocados!

2 ripe organic avocados
8 organic strawberries
2 tbsp Agave
2 tbsp cocoa powder

Wash and cut greens off of strawberries. Cut each avocado in half and remove the pit. Remove the avocado flesh and place in blender or food processor. Add the strawberries, the agave and the cocoa and blend or process on medium/high, mixing as needed for about 30-60 seconds (until smooth and well blended). Blend on high for an additional minute or so to make an even fluffier mousse. Place mousse in serving bowls and serve immediately or store in refrigerator for later use. This keeps in the refrigerator in an airtight container for up to one day.

Strawberry Shortcake Bars

Makes 20 bars
This is a fantastic version of strawberry shortcake that you can take with you anywhere!

1 cup raw sunflower seeds
1 cup pitted dates
14 nice size organic strawberries (will be a little more than 1 cup)
1 tsp vanilla extract
3 tbsp agave
3 tbsp water

Preheat oven to 180°. Spray cookie pan (15" x 10") with cooking spray and set aside.

Place all ingredients in blender or food processor and blend for 1-2 minutes. Mixture should be mixed well but still a little chunky. Carefully press mixture, evenly, into greased cookie pan, beginning in the center and working your way out to the edges. It may be helpful to wet your fingers with water so that the mixture doesn't stick to your hands.

Place in oven for 4-6 hours to dehydrate. When desired hardness is reached, remove from oven and let cool about 15 minutes. Cut into bars and let cool completely. Remove from cookie sheet and serve, or store in airtight container. These bars will keep in the refrigerator for up to two weeks.

Naturally Sweet Delicious Treats

5. SWEET ENDINGS AND TIDBITS

♥ Whenever possible, it is a good idea to use organic ingredients. Organic ingredients offer the least amount of contaminants and the highest nutritional value. I specify organic products in these recipes to ensure the highest level of nutrition in your baked goods.

♥ Whole grains are grains that have not been modified or refined. It is important to choose whole grains such as whole wheat flour, or unrefined oats. Whole grains are complex carbohydrates, which reduce the body's need for insulin to digest and process these treats. Whole grains also offer the body an abundance of nutrients as well as fiber.

♥ If nuts and/or seeds are not well tolerated, you may soak the raw nuts or seeds in a bowl of water for 4-12 hours prior to using. This activates enzymes in the raw nuts or seeds making them easier to digest. Make sure you rinse and drain well before using in your recipe. Soaking will only work for *raw* nuts and seeds.

♥ Potato starch is starch that has been extracted from potatoes. It is used in baking to retain moisture and texture. Potato starch can be found at some grocery stores and most health food stores.

♥ An *extract* is made from extracting natural flavors from a real food item such as vanilla beans, almonds, oranges etc... Extracts are the real deal! *Flavorings*, on the other hand are artificially created. Flavorings are chemical additives and are not natural. Make sure to purchase extracts such as *vanilla extract* and not *vanilla flavoring* when you are doing your wise shopping.

♥ Molasses is another natural sweetener. It is the syrupy byproduct of refining sugar. Molasses is loaded with vitamins and minerals such as calcium, manganese, copper and iron. Molasses has a robust flavor which may prove too strong for some baked goods, but compliments graham cookies nicely. Molasses is not a low glycemic food, but is not very sweet either. I enjoy the flavor of molasses and like to enhance the flavor of my baked goods and smoothies as well as add a nutritional boost by adding 1-2 tbsp. of blackstrap molasses.

♥ Raw honey has a history of healing benefits. It is loaded with nutritional enzymes that can heal the body in many ways. Raw honey has been known to cure cuts, heal acne, eczema, allergies, burns, arthritis, coughs, stress, yeast infections and more. Raw honey can be ingested or used topically. It can be used alone or mixed with other ingredients. Raw honey improves the immune system and helps to fight infection. Raw honey is truly a gift to health. Although all raw honey is good, keep in mind when purchasing raw honey that it is most beneficial to purchase raw honey that has been produced within a 20 mile radius of your home. This will ensure that you are getting all of the benefits of your local antibodies. Even though raw honey always retains its sweetness, the enzymes are destroyed at temperatures over 180°. Raw honey is the only honey I have in my pantry! (See note on page 11 regarding raw honey and infants under 12 months old)

♥ Chocolate is really a superfood! It is loaded with antioxidants and other nutrients that can help lower blood pressure and cholesterol, it acts as a natural anti-depressant, it can help reduce the risk of cancer, it is anti-inflammatory, it can increase longevity and it is a great food for the brain. I'm not talking about milk chocolate or the sweetened candy bars found on the shelves by the checkout counters - but rather a nice dark chocolate such as 70% to 85% cacao - preferable organic. The darker the chocolate the less sugar is contains. This healthy chocolate can come in the form of a solid block or bar, chocolate nibs, shavings or as a powder. Chocolate can boost your mood and your nutritional intake all at the same time! You can find dark, organic chocolate at some grocery stores and most health food stores.

"Live decently, fearlessly, joyously and don't forget that in the long run it is not the years in your life but the life in your years that counts!"
Adlai Stevenson

Trish Blascak

RECIPE INDEX

Trish Blascak

REFERENCES

Bittman, Mark, 2011, July 23, Sunday Review, The New York Times

Dictionary.com. (n.d.). *Poison.* ,
http://dictionary.reference.com/browse/poison

Essortment.com. (n.d.). *A Brief History on sugar, its values and production*.
  http://www.essortment.com/history-sugar-41718.html

Fallon, Sally. (2001). *Nourishing Traditions*. (Revised Second Edition). Washington, DC: NewTrends Publishing, Inc.

Mercola, Joseph & Pearsall, Kendra Degen. (2006). *Sweet Deception, Why Splenda, NutraSweet, and the FDA May Be Hazardous to Your Health.* Nashville, Tennessee: Thomas Nelson, Inc.

The American Academy of Pediatrics,
  http://www.aap.org

Trish Blascak